Makhlouf Dorsaf
Nahla Kechiche
Lassaad Sahnoun

Torsion of the spermatic cord on an ectopic testicle

AF551085

Makhlouf Dorsaf
Nahla Kechiche
Lassaad Sahnoun

Torsion of the spermatic cord on an ectopic testicle

Testicular torsion on an ectopic testicle in children

ScienciaScripts

Imprint
Any brand names and product names mentioned in this book are subject to trademark, brand or patent protection and are trademarks or registered trademarks of their respective holders. The use of brand names, product names, common names, trade names, product descriptions etc. even without a particular marking in this work is in no way to be construed to mean that such names may be regarded as unrestricted in respect of trademark and brand protection legislation and could thus be used by anyone.

Cover image: www.ingimage.com

This book is a translation from the original published under ISBN 978-620-6-72530-5.

Publisher:
Sciencia Scripts
is a trademark of
Dodo Books Indian Ocean Ltd. and OmniScriptum S.R.L publishing group

120 High Road, East Finchley, London, N2 9ED, United Kingdom
Str. Armeneasca 28/1, office 1, Chisinau MD-2012, Republic of Moldova, Europe
Printed at: see last page
ISBN: 978-620-8-31068-4

Copyright © Makhlouf Dorsaf, Nahla Kechiche, Lassaad Sahnoun
Copyright © 2024 Dodo Books Indian Ocean Ltd. and OmniScriptum S.R.L publishing group

CONTENTS

INTRODUCTION..2

OBJECTIVES...3

MATERIALS AND METHODS...................................4

RESULTS...6

DISCUSSION...20

CONCLUSION..35

BIBLIOGRAPHY...37

APPENDIXES..45

INTRODUCTION

The undescended testicle is a genital anomaly that refers to any anomaly in testicular migration, whether or not it is on the normal path of testicular descent.It is a complex, multifactorial disease [1]. Several hormonal, genetic and environmental factors are involved in its genesis and contribute to the recent increase in its incidence, particularly in industrialised countries. The seriousness of this condition lies in the immediate risk of torsion and the long-term risk of infertility and malignant transformation. The higher the position of the testicle, the greater the risk. This potential degeneration of the testicular gland into a seminoma occurs in adulthood between the ages of 30 and 40. Lowering the testicle into the bursa does not alter this risk.In addition to these major risks, there are the psychological consequences for patients with an absent, small or insufficiently descended testicle [3].

The clinical picture of a torsion of an ectopic testicle is unusual, exposing the patient to a high risk of delay in treatment. A number of issues remain controversial: pathophysiology, the role of imaging in diagnosis, the technique for fixation of the twisted testicle, the sutures to be used, the indication for orchiectomy and whether or not to fix the contralateral testicle.

OBJECTIVES

This is the context of our study project, in which we proposed to study the epidemiological, clinical and prognostic features of children operated on for torsion of an ectopic testicle.

MATERIALS AND METHODS

1-Type of study :

This is a retrospective study of 21 cases of torsion of an ectopic testicle in children operated on in the paediatric surgery department, Fatouma Bourguiba University Hospital, Monastir, over a 16-year period from January 2005 to July 2020.

2-Sampling :

The sample was based on exhaustive recruitment of all consulting patients whose diagnosis was torsion of an ectopic testicle.

* Inclusion criteria

All children operated on for torsion of an ectopic testicle in the paediatric surgery department of the CHU FBM

3-Measuring instrument :

Data were collected from medical records, operative reports and anatomopathological examination of orchiectomy specimens. Medical records and reports were analysed using a form that took the following elements into consideration: (appendix 1)

-Age

-Month of consultation

-Family and personal history and co-morbidities

-Symptomatology

-Physical examination

- paraclinical examinations

-surgical exploration and procedure performed

- Anatomopathological examination

post-operative follow-up

RESULTS

Our study included 21 patients operated on between January 2005 and January 2019 at the department of paediatric surgery CHU Fatouma Bourguiba Monastir for torsion on ectopic testis.

I- Clinical study: 1- Age :

The average age of the patients was 24 months (2 years), with extremes ranging from 11 days to 108 months (9 years).

Seventy-one point five percent of the children (71.5%) were infants aged between 1 month and 2 years.

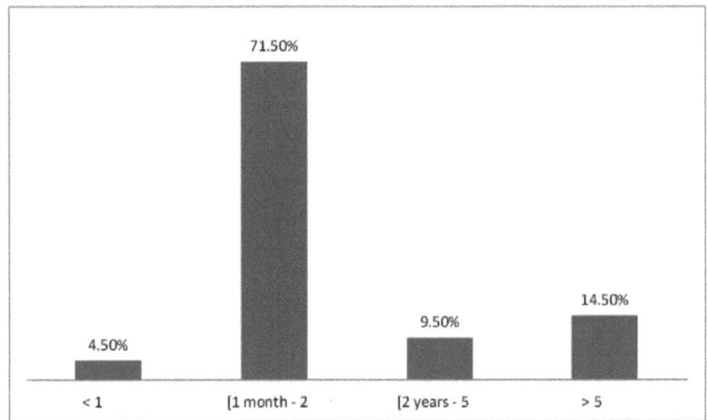

Figure 1: Breakdown of the study population by age group

2- Month of consultation :

Twenty-eight percent (28%) of the patients included in the study consulted a doctor in summer No statistically significant correlation between age and season of consultation (p=0.506).

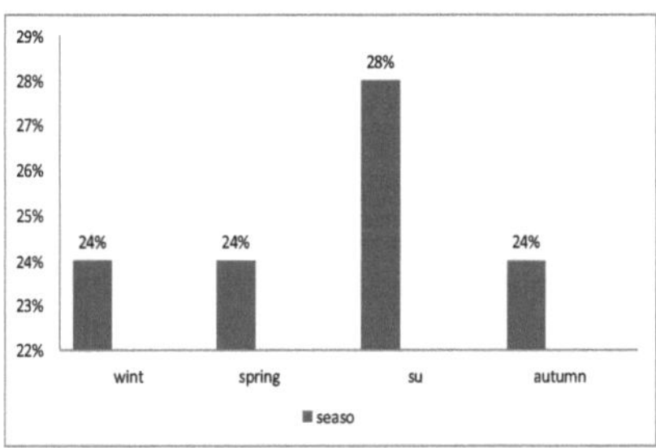

Figure 2: Breakdown of the study population by season of consultation

3- Family history :

In this study, no family history of cryptorchidism or testicular torsion was reported.

4- Personal history :

The most common personal histories were :

- Low birth weight (5%)
- Meningitis (9%)
- Maternal-foetal infection (5%)
- Neonatal respiratory distress (5%)
- Asthma (5%)
- Homolateral (5%) and bilateral (5%) inguinal hernia
- Patients known to have testicular ectopy 62% (unilateral in 38% and bilateral in 24%)

The following figure summarises the personal history

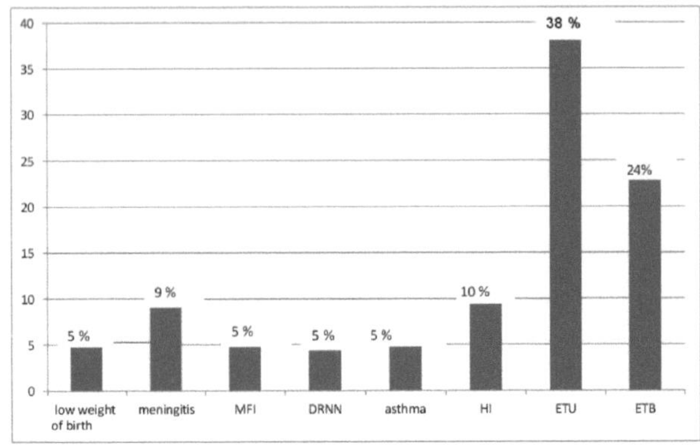

Figure 3: Breakdown of the study population by personal history

5- Comorbidities :

Co-morbidities were noted in 19% of children, in decreasing order of frequency:

- cerebral palsy (42%)
- epilepsy (9%),

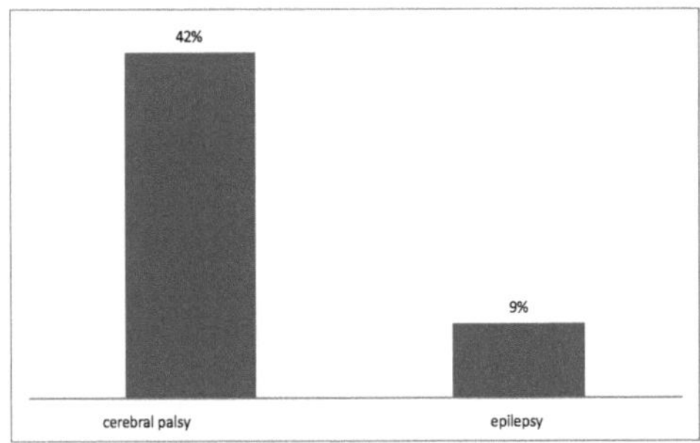

Figure 4: Percentage of patients with comorbidities in the study population

6- Reasons for consultation :

Inguinal swelling was the almost constant reason for consultation, present in 95% of cases. (Figure 5)

She was

- Associated with intense inguinal pain in **38%** of cases,
- local inflammatory signs in **9% of cases (Figure 6)**
- **5%** agitation

Inguinal pain alone was reported in only **5%** of cases.

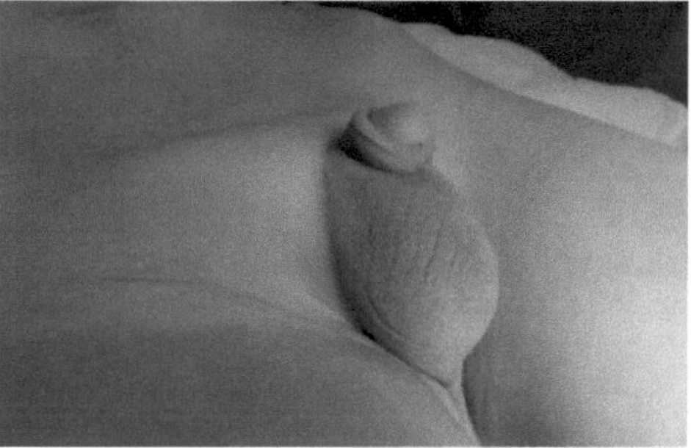

Figure 5: Right inguinal swelling with empty homolateral bursa

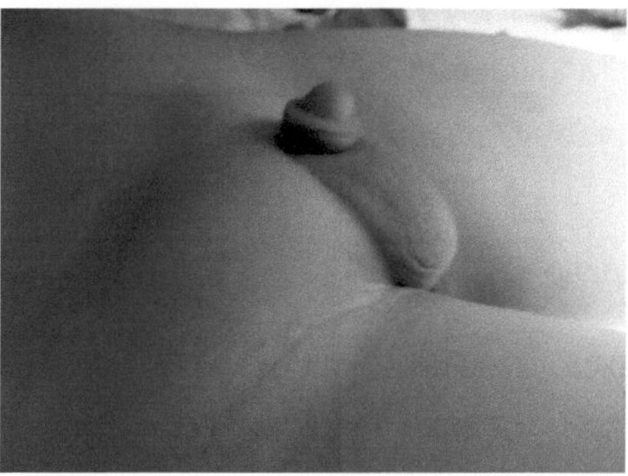

Figure 6: Right inguinal swelling with associated inflammatory signs

7- Duration of symptoms:

The average duration of symptoms was 31 hours, with a minimum of 12 hours and a maximum of 72 hours (fig 7). Sixty-six percent (66%) of patients consulted a doctor between 24 hours and 48 hours after the onset of symptoms.

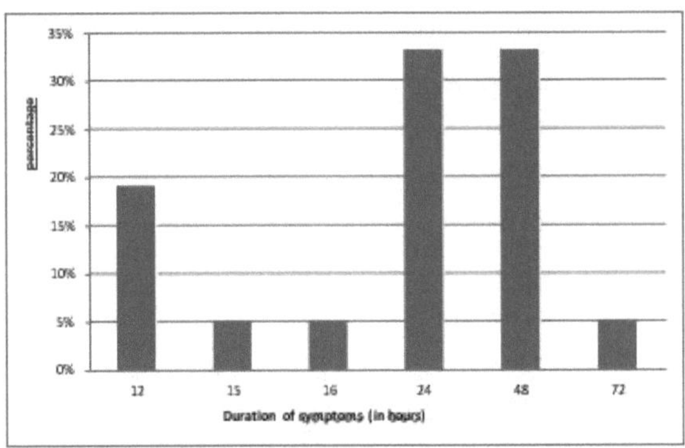

Figure 7: Breakdown of the study population by duration of symptoms

8- Associated signs :

Our results showed that the associated signs were essentially :

- Moderate fever ranging from 38.5 to 39 in 14%.
- Food vomiting in 9% of cases.

9- Physical examination :

Physical examination revealed a painful, intractable hard unilateral inguinal swelling with an empty homolateral bursa in 100% of cases; associated with local inflammatory signs (redness and heat) in 43% of cases.

10- Visit

In our study population, the affected testicle was left in 76% and right in 24% of cases (fig. 8).

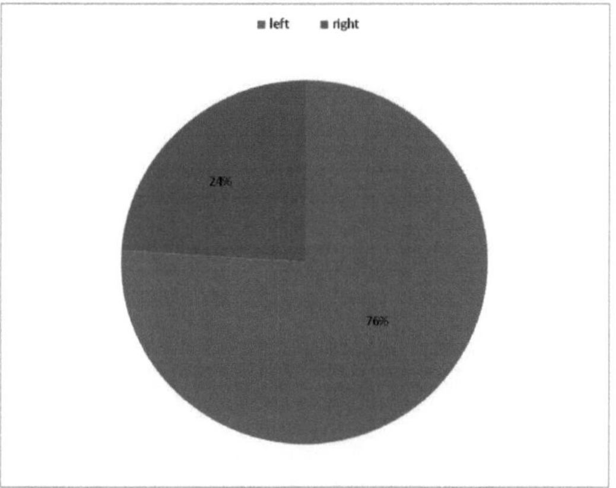

Figure 8: Distribution of the study population according to the side of the testicle affected

II-Paraclinical study :

1- Inguinal ultrasound :

Fifteen boys/21 had an inguinal ultrasound (71%): The ultrasound showed

An ectopic inguinal testicle with :

- A heterogeneous testicle in 52% of cases
- Peripheral vascularisation present in 20% of cases
- Reduced vascularity in 13% of cases
- Turns of coils (2 turns of coils) in 7
- A strangulated inguinal hernia with epiploic and testicular content with signs of testicular hypo-vitality was found in 7%.

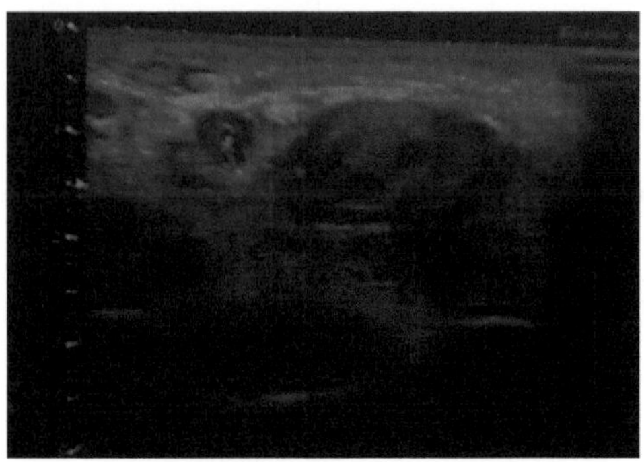

Figure 9 : Testis with heterogeneous echostructure and peripheral vascularisation

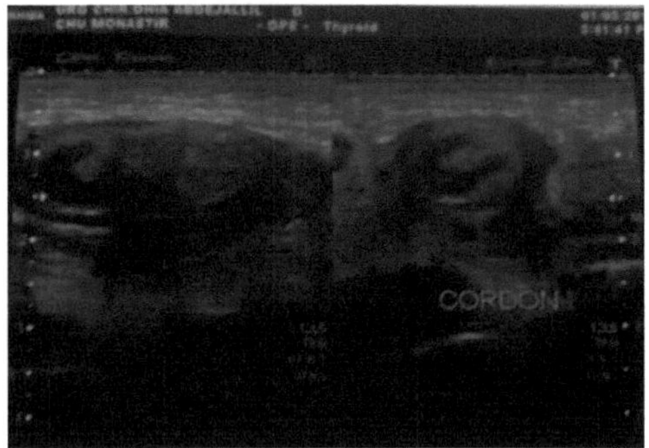

Figure 10: Ectopic testis with heterogeneous echostructure and reduced size

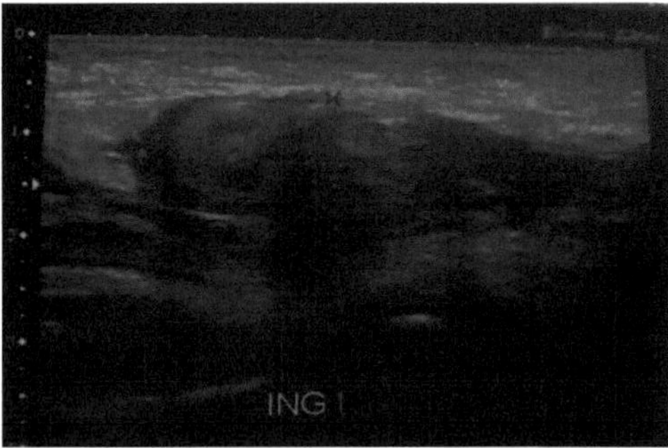

Figure 11 : Ectopic testis in the inguinal canal with heterogeneous echostructure and reduced size

2- Biology :

In our series, a biological check-up which was requested

- Was normal in 43% of cases
- Showed hyperleukocytosis in 43% of cases Results are shown in TableI

Table I: Biological results in the study population

	workforce	percentages
hyperleukocytosis	9	43 %
Hyperleukocytosis and high CRP	2	9 %
High CRP	1	5 %
Normal	9	43 %
TOTAL	21	100

III- Surgical exploration: 1- Approach :

In our series, exploration was performed in all cases by inguinal incision.

2- Exploration :

a- Type of torsion

The torsion was intra-vaginal in 71% of cases (fig 12).

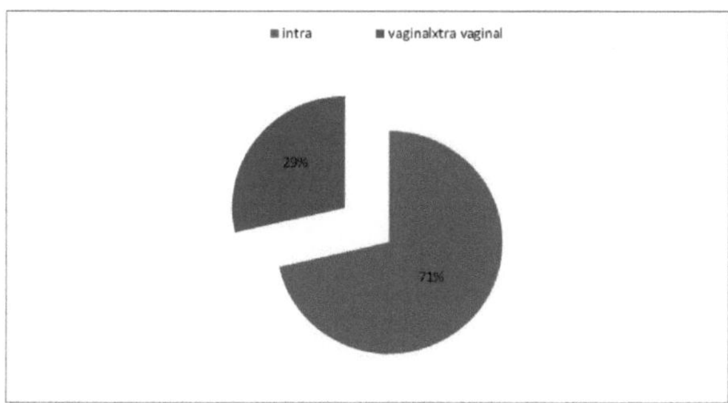

Figure 12: Location of the affected testicle according to surgical exploration b- Number of turns of the testicular torsion :

The number of turns of the testicular torsion was specified in 13 patients operated on in our series. In 38% of cases, the torsion consisted of two turns (fig.13).

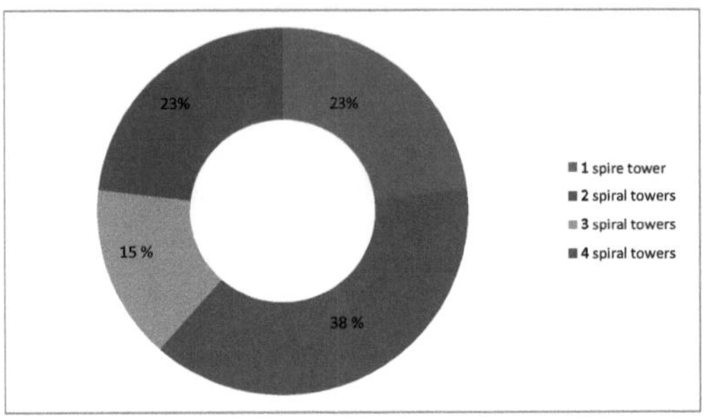

Figure 13: Number of turns c- Testicular vitality :

The intraoperative findings of our patients were as follows (fig.14):

- 86% black testicle
- 14% testicle Purplish blue

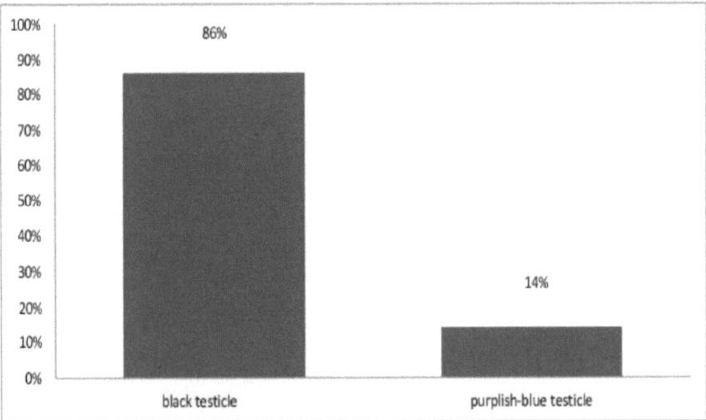

Figure 14: Intraoperative findings

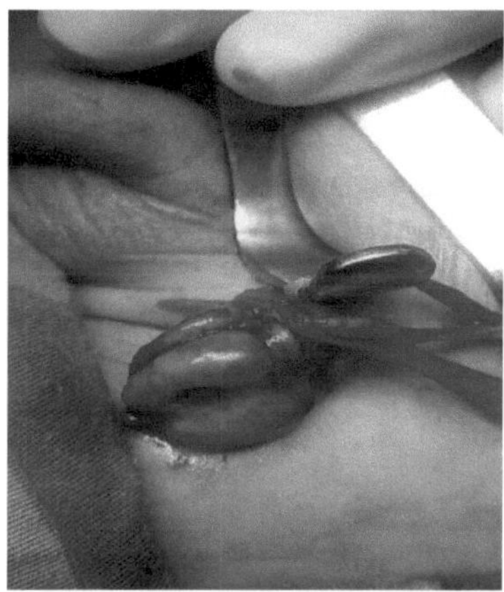

Figure 15: Spermatic cord torsion

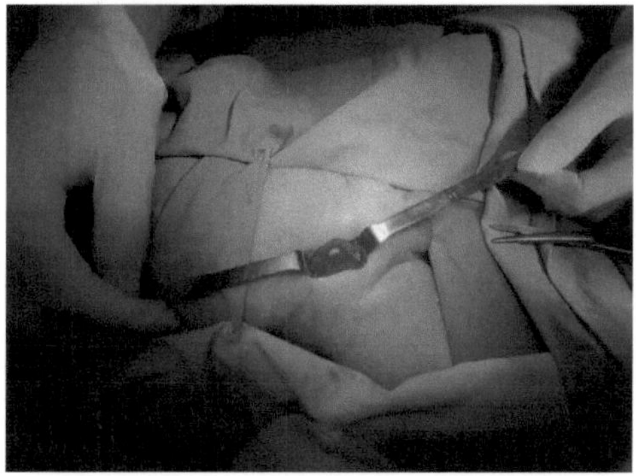

Figure 16: Edematous testicle

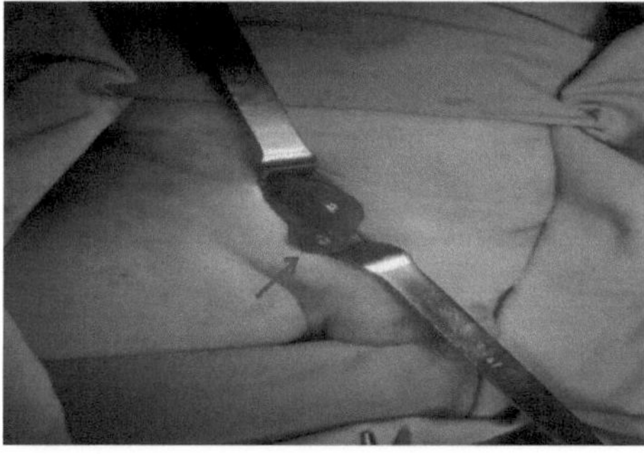

Figure 17: Torsion of the spermatic cord (arrow)

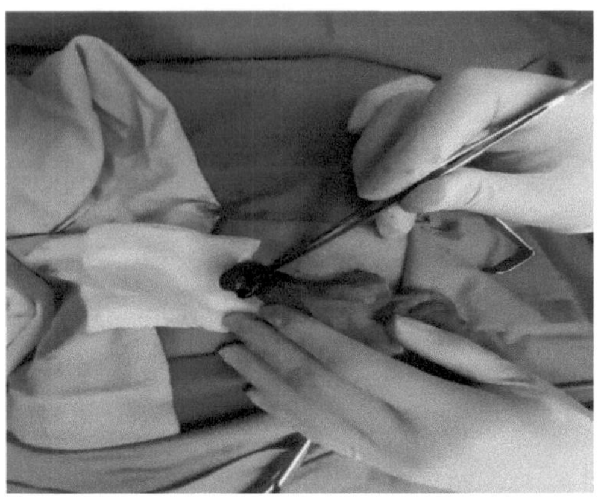

Figure 18: Blackish twisted ectopic testicle

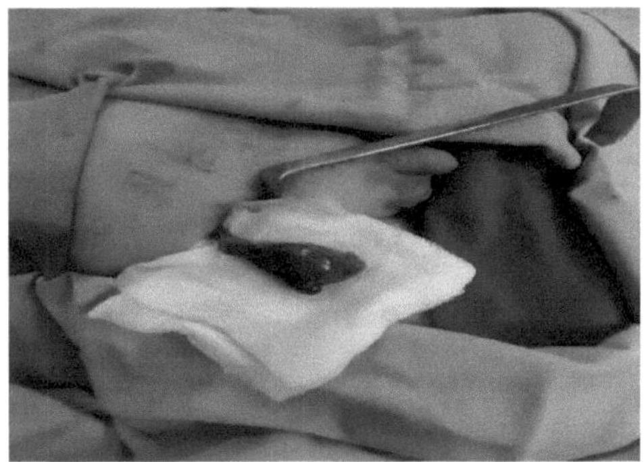

Figure 19: purplish-blue testicle after detorsion

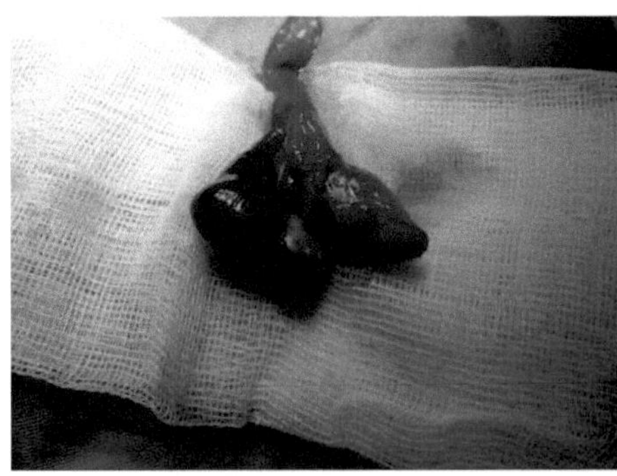

Figure 20: Ischaemic ectopic testicle not recoverable after detorsion

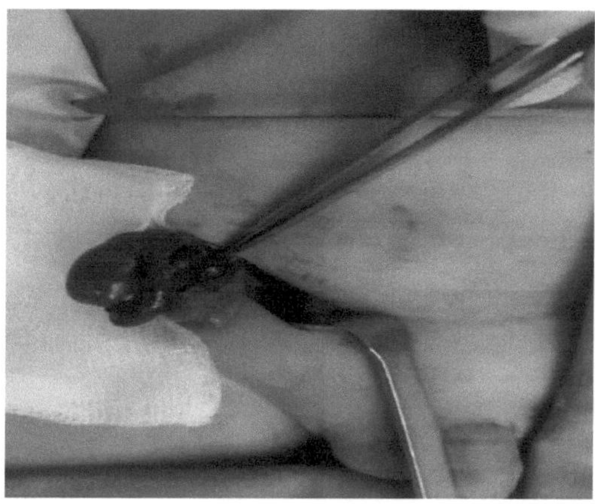

Figure 21: Black testicle with turn of spire (clamp)

IV- Surgical procedures:

1- procedure:

In our series :

- Orchidopexy was performed in 48% of patients (10 cases).
- Orchiectomy was performed in 52% of patients (11 cases) 2-

Contralateral testis :

Among our patients, 48% of the contralateral testicles were in place and did not undergo fixation, while 19% were ectopic and underwent lowering and orchidopexy at the same time.

Table II: Procedures performed according to the position of the contralateral testicle

Contralateral testis: position and gesture	percentage
in place, orchidopexy	19 %
in place, no fixing	48 %
ectopic, orchidopexy	19 %
ectopic, no fixation	14 %

V- Post-operative follow-up :

1-Immediate follow-up: Complications and length of hospital stay: No complications were noted postoperatively. Twenty patients were discharged 24 hours post-operatively. One child developed a viral fever and was discharged 96 hours post-operatively.

2-Long-term monitoring :

Follow-up over an average period of 1.8 months showed (11 patients were lost to follow-up, i.e. 43% of the study population):

- In the orchidopexy group: 3 patients had normal-sized testes (one of whom developed contralateral testicular torsion 4 months post-operatively and benefited from orchidopexy) and 2 patients had testicular atrophy.
- In the orchiectomy group: the contralateral testicles were all of normal size except in one patient where a testicle of reduced size was observed (the patient underwent an examination under GA showing: a hypoplastic testicle located at the root of the bursa and an orchidopexy was performed) (**tab n° III**).

Table III: Results of long-term follow-up of patients operated on for torsion of an ectopic testicle

<table>
<tr><th>Group</th><th colspan="2">Step back</th><th>Percentage</th></tr>
<tr><td rowspan="3">orchidopexy</td><td rowspan="2">Eutrophic testes</td><td>Contralateral testicular torsion</td><td>1 patient /5</td></tr>
<tr><td>No incidents</td><td>3 patients /5</td></tr>
<tr><td colspan="2">atrophic testicle</td><td>2 patients /5</td></tr>
<tr><td rowspan="3">orchiectomy</td><td colspan="2">Contralateral hypotrophy</td><td>1 patient / 5</td></tr>
<tr><td colspan="2">Eutrophic contralateral testes</td><td>4 patients/5</td></tr>
<tr><td colspan="2">Contralateral enlarged testes</td><td>0 patients/5</td></tr>
</table>

VI- Anatomopathology :

In this study, 11 patients underwent orchiectomy and anatomopathological examination showed: haemorrhagic necrosis in 100% of cases

DISCUSSION

Torsion of an implanted testicle is a fairly frequent occurrence in paediatric emergency departments. Its frequency varies in the literature, ranging from 20% to 30% [4-5]. It mainly affects children and adolescents, with an approximate incidence of 1 in 4000 men under the age of 25 [6]. In addition, torsion of an undescended testicle remains an exceptional condition; its incidence varies according to the series and depends on the choice and age of the study populations.

An undescended testicle is associated with a higher risk of torsion compared with a testicle in place. Williamson [2] estimates that the risk of torsion is 10 times higher in a cryptorchid testicle.Torsion of the spermatic cord is an extremely serious condition, and delay or misdiagnosis can lead to testicular ischaemia. This is why, in the event of any suspicion of testicular torsion, the patient must undergo surgical exploration as soon as possible, within the first 6 hours. No radiological examination should delay this procedure.

Given the risk of contralateral recurrence, prophylactic fixation of the contralateral testis at the same time as the operation is performed remains a subject of debate.In this study we report the cases of torsion on cryptorchid testicle operated in our service of paediatric surgery CHU Fatouma Bourguiba Monastir with an aim of better characterizing this pathology as well as facilitating the diagnosis in order to reduce the rate of orchiectomy.

I- Clinical study: 1-Incidence :

Testicular torsion is an uncommon condition, affecting 3.8% of men under the age of 18 [7]. Torsion of a cryptorchid testis remains a rare condition.

Diamopoulos et al [8] and Sauvat et al [9] found only 2 cases of torsion on an ectopic testicle in two series of 40 cases and 86 cases of testicular torsion.

2- Age

Torsion of a scrotal testicle is classically described in the literature as having a bimodal description with a double peak incidence mainly affecting newborns and young adolescents at the age of puberty [10]. The mean age of torsion of an ectopic testicle is comparable according to several studies to that of a testicle in place, it varied in the literature between 7.5 months and 10.8 years [11,12,13,14]. In our series, a peak of incidence was marked for infants aged between 1 month and 2 years (71.5%) with a mean age of 2 years.

3- Mechanisms and anatomical forms

The literature describes 2 mechanisms of testicular torsion independently of the location of the affected testicle (ectopic or in place): intravaginal and extravaginal. The intravaginal mechanism concerns the torsion of a testicle with a bell-shaped malformation: the tunica vaginalis covers the testicle, the epididymis and also part of the spermatic cord rather than being attached to them, creating a testicle in the tunica without attachment. This allows it to rotate freely around the axis of the strings. Extravaginal refers to cases without malformation, when the torsion occurs in the tunica vaginalis. [15,16]

Testicular torsion in children is classified according to age into 2 groups: perinatal torsion occurring from the prenatal period up to 1 month of life and non-neonatal torsion. In neonatal torsion: the spermatic cord, testicle and tunica vaginalis rotate together. This is therefore extravaginal torsion

[17]. In contrast, testicular torsion in infants and older children is mainly intravaginal [18]. The literature describes that approximately 90% of cases result from intravaginal torsion [19], in our series we also noted a clear predominance of intravaginal torsion among our patients with a percentage of 71%.

No difference was reported between the mechanism of torsion of an ectopic testicle compared with an implanted testicle. Torsion intravaginal remains by far the most common, regardless of testicular location, since infants are the age group most affected.

3- Month of consultation :

The relationship between the month of consultation and torsion of a cryptorchid testicle was not studied in the literature.

On the other hand, seasonal variation has been shown to contribute to torsion of a testis in place, with torsion being more common during the colder months especially in December and January [20].

Low ambient temperature can cause the cremasteric muscle to contract, leading to testicular torsion. [21]

Several studies have shown that testicular torsion has coincided with low ambient temperature (<15°) and low humidity [20, 21, 22, 23]. This is in contrast to the rate found in our study where 28% of patients consulted in summer. These results could have been affected by geographical differences and above all by the anatomical location of the testis.

3-Predisposing factors :

Torsion of a scrotal testis occurs mainly in children and young men with the following risk factors: an underlying bell flap deformity, an undescended testis, trauma and intermittent anterior torsion.[6] The risk factors for torsion of a scrotal testis are as follows On the other hand, several factors can predispose to torsion of a cryptorchid testicle:

-family :

A genetic predisposition has been suspected in several studies as a predictive factor for testicular torsion [24, 25, 26]. In our patients, no family history was found. This could be explained by the fact that this information was not sought during the interview.

-staff :

* testicular ectopia :

A history of unilateral or bilateral testicular ectopia has been reported in several studies [11, 27]. This is in good agreement with our results 62 % of our patients are known to have testicular ectopia.

*Prematurity and low birth weight:

According to several studies, the incidence of cryptorchidism in premature babies has been between 9% and 30%, which is much higher than in full-term babies (2.7%-5.9%) [28, 29]. This pathology is multiplied by 10 in premature babies and newborns with a low birth weight. [11, 15, 30, 31, 32] Taking this into account, ectopic testicular torsion is likely to occur in premature and low birth weight infants. Our patients were all born at term, but 5% of our patients had a low birth weight.

* Inguinal hernia:

The anomaly most frequently associated with undescended testis is inguinal hernia, a mechanical factor that impedes spontaneous migration of the testis [33]. In our series, an inguinal hernia was associated with 10% of cases. *necrotizing enterocolitis:

A study published in 2010 postulated that necrotising enterocolitis stimulates testicular torsion through intestinal inflammation [32]. It was thought that necrotising enterocolitis made the testes placed in the inguinal canal warmer and that the intestinal mucosa descended into the tunica. Consequently, testicular torsion in premature babies and newborns with ectopic testicles presenting intestinal infections remained highly probable.However, this notion was not explored during the interview.

*Other antecedents

Of our patients, 9% had meningitis, 5% had MFI, 5% had neonatal respiratory distress and 5% had asthma. Published studies did not report similar cases.

5- Comorbidities :

* Cerebral palsy (CP)

The prevalence of cryptorchidism in patients with BMI was estimated to be about 10 times higher than in the general population. [33]

The aetiopathogenesis remains poorly understood; several theories have been proposed: abnormal contraction or spasm of the cremasteric muscles causing torsion of the spermatic cord. This theory could be confirmed by the 53.8% incidence of cryptorchidism reported in BMI patients. Other publications have reported cases of ectopic testicular torsion in patients with spastic neuromuscular diseases. [16,34] In our series, 42% of patients had BMI and no spasmodic neuromuscular disease was reported.

* Epilepsy :

Several studies have reported a clear association between epilepsy and undescended testis in patients. Several diagnostic hypotheses have been discussed, the most relevant of which are chromosomal deletion disorders 6q *188 and dysfunctions. endocrine [35].

Epilepsy was also reported in 9% of our patients.

6- Reasons for consultation :

The main reason for consultation in cases of torsion of the ectopic testicle was inguinal swelling and/or pain. These two reasons were associated in 38% of cases in our study, and local inflammatory signs were associated with inguinal swelling in 9% of cases. Agitation was the most common symptom of pain in infants, and was the reason for consultation in 5% of cases. These data are in line with those of Naouar et al [11], where inguinal swelling was reported in 85% of cases, associated with local inflammatory signs in 15% and agitation isolated in an infant in 7%. In contrast to torsion of a testis in place where scrotal pain dominated the clinical picture associated with elevated position of the testis, scrotal swelling and changes in the scrotal skin [36, 37].

7- Duration of symptoms:

The mean time to progression in our study was 31 hours, with extremes of 12 hours and 72 hours. The mean duration of symptoms in the ochidopexy group was 21.4 hours and 38.4 hours in the orchiectomy group. These times were longer than those reported by Naouar et al [11]: the mean duration of symptoms was 14.5 with 6.5 h for the orchidopexy group and 21.2 h for the orchidectomy group.

This situation can be explained by parents' lack of awareness of the condition, but also by the predominance of frustrated or atypical forms.

8- Associated signs :

Our study showed that torsion of a cryptorchid testicle may be accompanied by fever in 14% of cases and by digestive signs such as vomiting in 9% of cases. These data are lower than those of Gharbi et al[31], where digestive symptoms were very significant and dominated the clinical picture in 40.6% of cases.

Several studies have also reported digestive signs: nausea and vomiting, which may be associated with torsion of an implanted testicle. Urinary signs such as dysuria may also be reported by patients [37].

9- Physical examination :

The physical signs in our study were obvious and included an intractable painful inguinal swelling with an empty homolateral bursa in all cases, associated with local inflammatory signs in 43% of cases. Our figures are comparable to those of Naouar et al*4 who also reported an inguinal swelling that was painful to palpation with an empty homolateral bursa in 92% of cases, with inflammatory signs in 15% of cases.

Sensitivity of the right iliac fossa on abdominal examination has been described in adult patients. [11, 38, 39]

During torsion of a testicle in place, the clinical examination is much more obvious, and plays a major role in the investigation of acute scrotum according to a review of the literature [40]. It revealed: an absent or pathological cremasteric reflex in 80%, an abnormal position of the testicle in 64%, diffuse scrotal sensitivity to palpation in 94.8%, scrotal oedema in 68.3% or testicular oedema in 66% and scrotal erythema in 45.2%. Torsion of a scrotal testicle can be assessed using the TWIST score (Testicular Workup for Ischemia and Suspected Torsion). The scoring is as follows: testicular swelling (2 points), hard testicle (2 points), absent cremasteric reflex (1 point), nausea and vomiting (1 point) and high-level testicle (1 point). A score of 0 is predictive of non-torsion, and a score of 6 or 7 is highly predictive of testicular torsion [41]. The use of this score is limited to torsion of an established testis.

10- Coté :

Torsion of the left testicle is estimated to be 2 times more frequent whatever the position of the affected testicle because the left cord is longer. [11, 31, 39, 42,43 ,44] Our series also showed a predominance of the left side in 76 of cases.

II- Paraclinical study :

1- Ultrasound and abnormalities described :

Ultrasound coupled with Doppler has been proven to be the first-line imaging modality in cases of suspected torsion of an ectopic testicle or in cases of acute scrotum. It is used to confirm the diagnosis and predict the functional prognosis of the testicle [45]. However, its sensitivity is only 69.2% and its specificity 100% in the case of acute scrotum. [46] and only 13 to 17% in the case of non-palpable ectopic testis.[47] Some authors even consider that ultrasound exploration and possibly Doppler examination contribute little in children and that this examination only delays surgical treatment [48]. This ultrasound looked for coils and allowed us to conclude that there was no vascularisation. Visualisation of vascularisation is not a pathognomonic sign of spermatic cord torsion.

Visualisation of coils is much more reliable with a sensitivity of 99% compared with 76% in the series by Kalfa et al [49].

Abdominal ultrasound is considered to be unreliable for the diagnosis of ectopic testicular torsion: Nadav [50] presented three patients with a history of ectopy who were admitted to emergency due to agitation and painful inguinal mass. In two patients Doppler diagnosed an incarcerated hernia, but surgical exploration revealed torsion of the undescended testes with no evidence of an incarcerated hernia. In the third case, Doppler ultrasound demonstrated testicular torsion, but surgery revealed an incarcerated inguinal hernia with no evidence of testicular torsion.Hence the need for clinicians to be wary, as the diagnosis can be difficult and the results of Doppler ultrasound can be misleading. Only one of our 15 patients who underwent Doppler ultrasound showed a strangulated inguinal hernia with epiploic and testicular content, with signs of testicular hypo-vitality, which was then invalidated intraoperatively. The sonographic features of testicular torsion in neonates have been divided according to Traubici et al [51] into three types: type I included a marked increase in size of the affected testis with heterogeneity, with no detectable Doppler sign; type II showed a testis of normal size with heterogeneity and peripheral hyperechogenicity; and type III consisted of a testis markedly decreased in size and areas of hyperechogenicity scattered throughout the testis. Type I was associated with testicular torsion in the acute phase, and types II and III reflect the later phases of progressive parenchymal atrophy. In our series there was no specific ultrasound appearance that predicted testicular functional prognosis.

It is important to note that the characteristic sign of testicular torsion on ultrasound is the absence of testicular blood flow or swirl signs (torsion of the spermatic cord). It should not be forgotten that Doppler ultrasound remains an operator-dependent

examination, with highly variable sensitivity. Therefore, if there is any doubt, imaging should not delay surgical exploration.

2- Biology :

The literature gives no importance to the biological work-up, which is often unremarkable. Our results were also consistent: the work-up was normal in 43% of our patients.

III- Surgical exploration: 1-Access :

The inguinal approach was the rule in cases of torsion of an ectopic testicle. A scrotal incision is indicated in cases of torsion of a testicle in place.

2- Prognostic factors :

Several studies have stated that the degree of ischaemia was directly dependent on the duration, degree of rotation and thickness of the spermatic cord. [42,52]

Thicker cords lead to the formation of longer helices with impaired blood flow than thinner cords for the same degree of torsion. [52]

Testicular torsion salvage rates have been estimated to range from 90-100% if detorsion occurs within 6 hours of symptom onset but decrease to 20% after 12 hours and from 10% to 0% if delayed for more than 24 hours. [53]

Bartsch et al [54] have reported that irreversible ischaemic damage to the testicular parenchyma can begin as early as 4 hours after cord occlusion.

Bearing in mind the potentially catastrophic consequences of delay or misdiagnosis, the current approach is as follows: any patient presenting with a possible testicular torsion should undergo surgical exploration as soon as possible, within the first 6 hours. No radiological examination should delay this procedure. Ultrasound should only be offered if it can be performed without delaying surgery, or alternatively to confirm another diagnosis.

3- Number of turns of the testicular torsion :

Experimental studies have shown that torsion of the spermatic cord <360° may not compromise testicular blood flow [55,56] In our series, we had 61% of patients with 1 to 2 loosely packed coils (<360°), which explains the number of testicles saved despite the average evolution time of 31 hours.

4- Intraoperative findings :

Gharbi et al [31] reported in their series that 60% of the testicles were obviously necrotic; this finding was also found in our series with a percentage of 86%.In the operative report, we must specify the duration of evolution (major prognostic factor) and the thickness of the cord, the number of turns, the direction and degree and the appearance of the testicle (use a standardised scale for the degree of bruising).

IV- Surgical procedures:

V- 1- procedure:

Surgery consists firstly of exploring the affected side, and if the diagnosis is confirmed, detorsion of the testicle, and if revascularisation is satisfactory, fixation of the testicle after it has been lowered. Orchiectomy is performed if the testicle is clearly necrotic. In intermediate cases, the therapeutic decision is difficult to make. Comadoe et al [57] have studied 3 parameters which may facilitate the therapeutic choice: the evolution of symptoms lasting more than 10 hours, the absence of flow blood flow à ultrasound Doppler and the absence bleeding after incision of the tunicaalbuginea.Theseparameters may point towards orchiectomy. Naouar et al [11] reported a mean duration of symptoms at the time of surgery of 6.5 hours in cases treated with orchidopexy and 21.2 hours in the orchiectomy group.However, our results showed longer durations: the average duration in the orchidopexy group was 22 hours and 39 hours in the orchidectomy group. A difference in the age ranges of the study populations could be at the root of this difference. The type of fixation has been widely debated in the literature [58], as many recurrences have been described [59]. Several methods have been described and are currently used for testicular fixation, such as suture fixation of the testicle or creation of a dartos pocket.The use of absorbable sutures accompanied recurrence in most cases.

It is interesting to note that the scrotal pouch and vaginal eversion with dartos fixation using non-absorbable sutures could be superior to other known techniques and looks promising. Orchiectomy is indicated in cases where symptoms have progressed for more than 10 hours, there is no vascularisation on echo-Doppler and there is no bleeding after incision of the albuginea.

2- Contralateral testis :

Although prophylactic fixation of the contralateral testis is recommended by the majority of authors to reduce the risk of contralateral recurrence and preserve fertility for patients, a recent study [60] suggested that performing this procedure after torsion of an established testis did not appear to provide any benefit and was associated with a higher rate of postoperative complications. The literature recommends 2 different options; fixation of the contralateral testis is performed either in the same operative time or in a second time [13]In our study, 38% of patients underwent contralateral prophylactic orchidopexy at the same time as the operation.

Contralateral orchidopexy is not recommended. Long-term sterility has been described and it is also associated with a high rate of post-operative complications. Orchidopexy should be performed on a limited scale, and after informing the patient of the risks and potential benefits.

VI- Post-operative follow-up: 1-Immediate follow-up :

No complications have been reported in the literature during the postoperative period, which is the same for our results.
2- Long-term monitoring :

After 2 years of follow-up in 6 patients who had undergone orchidopexy Gharbi et al. [31] reported: 1 case of normal testicle size, 3 cases of hypotrophy and 2 cases of testicular atrophy. Our results showed normal sized testes in 3 of 5 patients who had orchidopexy compared with 2 cases of testicular atrophy. Contralateral testicular torsion was noted in one patient. No study has looked at the long-term impact on patients' fertility. However, deleterious effects on the sperm count, in particular the creation of anti-sperm antibodies, have been reported in the long term [1].

VII- Anatomopathology :

Torsion of the spermatic cord reduces the blood supply to the testicles, leading to haemorrhage, infarction and necrosis. Numerous studies have shown that testicular infarction begins within the first 2 hours after the onset of spermatic cord torsion, irreversible damage occurs after 6 hours and complete infarction develops after 24 hours [61]. In our series, 100% of pathological examinations showed haemorrhagic necrosis. No tumour testis was noted in our study.These results were close to those of Naouar et al [11] and Gharbi et al [12].[32] who found haemorrhagic testicular infarcts and necrosis on anatomopathological examination of the majority of excised testes, with a testicular tumour found only in one adult patient.Long-term follow-up of these patients (fertility, psychological repercussions and testicular ultrasound appearance) would appear to be of interest in order to draw conclusions about the value of orchidopexy in the case of an ischaemic testicle.

Table IV: Comparison between duration of symptoms and intraoperative appearance in the orchiectomy group

patients	Duration of symptoms (in hours)	Intraoperative aspect
1	48 hours	Necrotic testis
2	48 hours	Necrotic testis
3	24 hours	Necrotic testis
4	24 hours	Necrotic testis
5	48 hours	Purplish-blue testicle
6	24 hours	Necrotic testis
7	72 hours	Necrotic testis
8	48 hours	Necrotic testis
9	48 hours	Necrotic testis
10	24 hours	Necrotic testis
11	24 hours	Purplish-blue testicle

Table V: Duration of symptoms, intraoperative findings and long-term outcome in the orchidopexy group

Patients	Development time of symptoms (in hours)	Intraoperative observation	Long-term trends
1	12 hours	Blackish testicle	normal-sized testicle with contralateral testicular torsion (after 5 months)
2	4 p.m.	Blackish testicle	Atrophic testis
3	12 hours	Testis blackish	Lost from sight
4	24 hours	Blackish testicle	Lost from sight
5	12 hours	Blackish testicle	Lost from sight
6	12 hours	Blackish testicle	Testis of normal size
7	3 p.m.	Blackish testicle	Lost from sight
8	48 hours	Purplish-blue testicle	Lost from sight
9	48 hours	Blackish testicle	Atrophic testis
10	24 hours	Blackish testicle	Lost from sight

CONCLUSION

Torsion of the spermatic cord on an undescended testicle is a rare condition. Mechanical strangulation of the spermatic cord results in compression of the venous and arterial elements, rapidly leading to complete and irreversible necrosis of the testicle due to ischaemia. This is the context of our study, in which we propose to assess the prevalence of testicular torsion in order to better characterise this pathology and thus reduce the rate of orchiectomy.To meet these objectives we conducted a retrospective study, we included 21 cases of undescended testicular torsion, which were operated in the department of pediatric surgery CHU Fatouma Bourguiba Monastir. This study covers a 16-year period from January 2005 to July 2020. At the end of our work, the following findings emerge:Our patients ranged in age from 11 days to 9 years, with an average age of 2 years and a peak in the age range 1 month to 2 years. Sixty-two percent (62%) of patients were followed up for ectopic testis and 42% of patients had cerebral palsy. Inguinal swelling was the reason for consultation in 95% of cases, associated with inguinal pain in 38% of cases. Clinical examination revealed a hard inguinal swelling that was painful and irreducible to palpation, with an empty homolateral bursa in all patients, associated with local inflammatory signs in 43%. The affected testicles were 76% left. The diagnosis of torsion of an ectopic testicle was made by Doppler ultrasound in 15 patients and was confirmed by surgical exploration in all patients. The mean duration of symptoms was 22 hours in the orchidopexy group and 39 hours in the orchidectomy group. Long-term follow-up of orchidopexy patients showed testicular atrophy in 2 patients. At the end of this work, it appears that the torsion of an ectopic testicle in children is an infrequent but serious pathology which involves the functional prognosis of the testicles. It should be suspected in any child with a history of testicular ectopia who presents with painful inguinal swelling. Doppler ultrasonography remains an operator-dependent examination with variable sensitivity, and should only be requested in the event of a diagnosis. Under no circumstances should it delay surgical management, which should take place within the first 6 hours. Surgical exploration often reveals intravaginal torsion, the pathophysiological mechanism of which is a bell-shaped malformation. Orchidopexy is indicated in the presence of a viable testicle, the technique The most recommended method of fixation is vaginal eversion with dartos fixation using non-absorbable sutures. Orchiectomy remains the last resort when these 3 parameters are met: symptoms evolve for more than 10 hours, there is no blood flow on Doppler ultrasound and there is no bleeding after incision of the tunica albuginea.Fixation of the contralateral testicle is strongly discouraged because of postoperative complications and the risk of long-term infertility. Long-term follow-up is important to assess the condition of the operated testicle. Long-term results are to be judged on the trophicity of the detoriated testicle as well as on the fertility of these patients.

BIBLIOGRAPHY

1- Karl J., Capel B., Dev Biol Sertoli cells of the mouse testis originate from the coelomic epithelium. 998 Nov 15; 203(2): 323-33.

2- Williamson RC. Torsion of the testis and allied conditions. Br J Surg. 1976 Jun;63(6):465-76. doi: 10.1002/bjs.1800630618. PMID: 6106.

3- Cummings J.M., Boullier J.A., Sekhon D., Bose K. Adult testicular torsion J Urol 2002 ; 167 : 2109-2110

4- Valla JS, Steyaert H, Colomb F, Ginier C. Management of acute swollen scrotum in children. [Management of acute swollen scrotum in children.] Ann.Chir. 1998;52(10):1033-7.

5- Cavusoglu YH, Karaman A, Karaman I, Erdogan D, Aslan MK, Varlikli O, et al. Acute scrotum -- etiology and management. Indian J.Pediatr. 2005; Mar;72(3):201-3.

6- Palmer LS, Palmer JS. Management of abnormalities of the external genitalia in boys. In: Wein AJ, Kavoussi LR, Partin AW, et al, editors. Campbell-Walsh urology. 11th ed. Philadelphia: Elsevier; 2016. p. 3384-97

7- Lee C Zhao 1, Timothy B Lautz, Joshua J Meeks, Max Maizels. Pediatric testicular torsion epidemiology using a national database: incidence, risk of orchiectomy and possible measures toward improving the quality of care. J Urol. 2011 Nov;186(5):2009-13

8- Dimopoulos C, Giannopoulos A, Doïkas J, Ntoutsias A. Unusual presentation of testicular torsion. A review of 40 cases. Eur Urol. 1976;2(4):179-81. doi: 10.1159/000471998. PMID: 1009973.

9- Sauvat F, Hennequin S, Ait Ali Slimane M, Gauthier F. An age for testicular torsion? [Age for testicular torsion?] Arch Pediatr. 2002

Dec;9(12):1226-9. French. doi: 10.1016/s0929-693x(02)00112-4. PMID: 12536102.

10- Cuckow PM, Frank JD. Torsion of the testis. BJU Int. 2000 Aug;86(3):349-53. doi: 10.1046/j.1464-410x.2000.00106.x. PMID: 10930945.

11- Naouar S, Braiek S, El Kamel R. Testicular torsion in undescended testes: a persistent challenge. Asian J Urol . 2017; 4 (2): 111-115. doi: 10.1016 / j.ajur.2016.05.007

12- Gnassingbe K et al . les torsions du cordon spermatique chez l'enfant .African Journal of urology . vol 15.2009 .263-267.

13- Dorit Zilberman, Yael Inbar, Zehava Heyman, Danny Shinhar, Ron Bilik, Itamar Avigad, Paul Jonas, Jacob Ramon, Yoram Mor, Torsion of the Cryptorchid Testis-Can It be Salvaged?,The Journal of Urology, Volume 175, Issue 6, 2006, 2287-2289

14- Boettcher M, Bergholz R, Krebs TF, Wenke K, Aronson DC. Clinical predictors of testicular torsion in children. Urology. 2012 Mar;79(3):670-4. doi: 10.1016/j.urology.2011.10.041. PMID: 22386422.

15- Candocia FJ, Sack-Solomon K. An infant with testicular torsion in the inguinal canal. Pediatr Radiol. 2003 Oct;33(10):722-4. doi: 10.1007/s00247- 003-0984-8. Epub 2003 Aug 22. PMID: 12937868.

16- Schultz KE. Walker J. Testicular Torsion in Undescended Testes. Ann Emerg Med 1984;13:7.

17- Baglaj M, Carachi R. Neonatal bilateral testicular torsion: a plea for emergency exploration. J Urol 2007;177:2296-9

18- Caesar RE, Kaplan GW. Incidence of the bell-clapper deformity in anautopsy series. Urology 1994;44:114-6

19- Toft P, Nikolajsen IL. Torsion of intra-abdominal non-malignant testis. A case report. Acta Chir Scand. 1986 Jan;152:77-8. PMID: 3953225

20- Hoshino H, Abe T, Watanabe H, Katsuoka Y, Kawamura N. Correlation between atmospheric temperature and testicular torsion. Hinyokika Kiyo. 1993;39(11):1031-1033. discussion 1033-1034. Japanese

21- Shukla RB, Kelly DG, Daly L, Guiney EJ. Association of cold weather with testicular torsion. Br Med J (Clin Res Ed) 1982;285(6353):1459-1460

22- Molokwu CN, Somani BK, Goodman CM. Outcomes of scrotal exploration for acute scrotal pain suspicious of testicular torsion: a consecutive case series of 173 patients. BJU Int. 2011 Mar;107(6):990-3. doi: 10.1111/j.1464-410X.2010.09557.x. Epub 2010 Sep 21. PMID: 21392211.

23- Srinivasan AK, Freyle J, Gitlin JS, Palmer LS. Climatic conditions and the risk of testicular torsion in adolescent males. J Urol. 2007 Dec;178(6):2585-8; discussion 2588. doi: 10.1016/j.juro.2007.08.049. Epub 2007 Oct 22. PMID: 17945301.

24- Thorup J, Cortes D, Petersen BL. The incidence of bilateral cryptorchidism is increased and the fertility potential is reduced in sons born to mothers who have smoked during pregnancy. J Urol. 2006 Aug;176(2):734-7. doi: 10.1016/j.juro.2006.03.042. PMID: 16813933.

25- Shteynshlyuger A, Yu J. Familial testicular rtorsion: a meta analysis suggests inheritance. J Pediatr Urol 2013;9:683-90.

26- Pierik FH, Burdorf A, Deddens JA, Juttmann RE, Weber RF. Maternal and paternal risk factors for cryptorchidism and hypospadias: a case-control study in newborn boys. Environ Health Perspect. 2004

Nov;112(15):1570-6. doi: 10.1289/ehp.7243. PMID: 15531444; PMCID: PMC1247623.

27- Docimo SG, Silver RI, Cromie W. The undescended testicle: diagnosis and management. Am Fam Physician. 2000;62:2037-44, 2047-8

28- Pillai SB, Besner GE. Pediatric testicular problems. Pediatr Clin North Am. 1998;45:813.

29- Scorer CG. The descent of the testis. Arch Dis Child. 1964;39:605-9.

30- Bartley G. Cilento, Samir S. Najjar, Anthony Atala, Cryptorchidism and Testicular Torsion,Pediatric Clinics of North America,Volume 40, Issue 6,1993, 1133-1149.

31- Gharbi M, Amri N, Chambeh W, Braiek S, Kamel RE. Torsion of cryptorchid testis. Can Urol Assoc J. 2010;4(6):393-396.

32- Jung YJ, Chung JM. Testicular torsion in the inguinal region in an extremely low birth weight infant. Korean J Pediatr. 2010;53(9):852-854. doi:10.3345/kjp.2010.53.9.852

33- Barthold JS, Wintner A, Hagerty JA, Rogers KJ, Hossain MJ. Cryptorchidism in Boys With Cerebral Palsy Is Associated With the Severity of Disease and With Co-Occurrence of Other Congenital Anomalies. Front Endocrinol (Lausanne). 2018;9:151. Published 2018 Apr 16. doi:10.3389/fendo.2018.00151

34- Ito T, Matsui F, Fujimoto K, Matsuyama S, Yazawa K, Matsumoto F, Shimada K. Acquired undescended testis and possibly associated testicular torsion in children with cerebral palsy or neuromuscular disease. J Pediatr Urol. 2018 Oct;14(5):402-406. doi: 10.1016/j.jpurol.2018.08.015. Epub 2018 Aug 23. PMID: 30219308.

35- Thapa LJ, Pokharel BR, Paudel R, Rana PV. Association of seizure, facial dysmorphism, congenital umbilical hernia and undescended testes. Kathmandu Univ Med J (KUMJ). 2012 Jan-Mar;10(37):91-3. doi: 10.3126/kumj.v10i1.6924. PMID: 22971872.

36- Srinivasan A, Cinman N, Feber KM, Gitlin J, Palmer LS. History and physical examination findings predictive of testicular torsion: an attempt to promote clinical diagnosis by house staff. J Pediatr Urol. 2011 Aug;7(4):470-4. doi: 10.1016/j.jpurol.2010.12.010. Epub 2011 Mar 30. PMID: 21454130.

37- Sharp VJ, Kieran K, Arlen AM. Testicular torsion: diagnosis, evaluation, and management. Am Fam Physician. 2013 Dec 15;88(12):835-40. PMID: 24364548.

38- Ueno K , Hayashi H, Oohama K, AsanoS . Missed Torsion of an Undescended Testis Detected with Testicular Imaging. Journal of Nuclear Medicine June 1987, 28 (6) 1061.

39- Plitt DC, Fotos JS, Hulse MA, Neutze JA. Testicular ascent as a mechanism for intra-abdominal torsion. Radiol Case Rep. 2015;5(2):299. Published 2015 Nov 6. doi:10.2484/rcr.v5i2.299

40- Lafitte A, Joseph JM , Gehr M. Testicular torsion: a challenge for the primary care physician. Literature review and meta-analysis of diagnostic devices. Lausanne, September 2016.

41- Sheth KR, Keays M, Grimsby GM, Granberg CF, Menon VS, DaJusta DG, Ostrov L, Hill M, Sanchez E, Kuppermann D, Harrison CB, Jacobs MA, Huang R, Burgu B, Hennes H, Schlomer BJ, Baker LA. Diagnosing Testicular Torsion before Urological Consultation and Imaging: Validation of the TWIST Score. J Urol. 2016 Jun;195(6):1870-6. doi: 10.1016/j.juro.2016.01.101. Epub 2016 Feb 2. PMID: 26835833.

42- RINGDAHL.E. Testicular Torsion. Am Fam Physician. 2006 Nov

15;74(10):1739-1743.

43 -ein SH ET AL. "Torsion of an Undescended Intraabdominal Benign Testicular Teratoma." The Journal of Urology, 139(2), p. 444

44- Even L, Abbo O, Le Mandat A, Lemasson F, Carfagna L, Soler P et al. Spermatic cord torsion in children: impact of mode of consultation on management delay and orchiectomy rate. Arch Pediatr. 2013; 20: 364-368

45- Cavusoglu YH, Karaman A, Karaman I, Erdogan D,Aslan MK, Varlikli O, et al. Acute scrotum -- etiology and management. Indian J.Pediatr. 2005; Mar;72(3):201-3.

46- Lam WW, Yap TL, Jacobsen AS, Teo HJ. Colour Doppler ultrasonography replacing surgical exploration for acute scrotum: Myth or reality? Pediatr.Radiol. 2005;Jun;35(6):597-600.

47- RAMBEAUD J.J., GREATOREX R.A.: Torsion of the testis and its appendages. Encylop. Med. Chir., Nephrol. Urol, 1991, 18622-A-10

48- Van Glabeke E, Khairouni A, Larroquet M, Audry G, Gruner M. Spermatic cord torsion in children. [Spermatic cord torsion in children.] Prog.Urol.1998; Apr;8(2):244-8.

49- Kalfa N, Veyrac C, Lopez M, Lopez C, Maurel A, Kaselas C, et al. Multicenter assessment of ultrasoundof the spermatic cord in children with acute scrotum. J.Urol. 2007; Jan;177(1):297,301; discussion 301.

50- Nadav Slijper MD et al. Critical Validation of Ultrasound Doppler in the Diagnosis of Torsion of Undescended Testis.IMAJ. February 2007.vol9.99- 101

51- Traubici J, Daneman A, Navarro O, Mohanta A, Garcia C.Testicular torsion in neonates and infants: sonographic features in 30 patients. AJR

Am J Roengenol 2003;180:1143-5.

52- Bentley DF, Ricchiuti DJ, Nasrallah PF, McMahon DR. Spermatic cord torsion with preserved testis perfusion: initial anatomical observations. J Urol. 2004 Dec;172(6 Pt 1):2373-6. doi: 10.1097/01.ju.0000145527.08591.27. PMID: 15538271.

53- Cattolica EV, Karol JB, Rankin KN, Klein RS. High testicular salvage rate in torsion of the spermatic cord. The Journal of Urology. 1982 Jul;128(1):66-68. DOI: 10.1016/s0022-5347(17)52758-5.

54- Bartsch G, Frank S, Marberger H, Mikuz G. Testicular torsion: late results with special regard to fertility and endocrine function. J Urol. 1980 Sep;124(3):375-8. doi: 10.1016/s0022-5347(17)55456-7. PMID: 6776291

55- Bader TR, Kammerhuber F, Herneth AM. Testicular blood flow in boys as assessed at color Doppler and power Doppler sonography. Radiology. 1997 Feb;202(2):559-64. doi: 10.1148/radiology.202.2.9015090. Erratum in: Radiology 1997 May;203(2):580. PMID: 9015090.

56- Lee FT Jr, Winter DB, Madsen FA, Zagzebski JA, Pozniak MA, Chosy SG, Scanlan KA. Conventional color Doppler velocity sonography versus color Doppler energy sonography for the diagnosis of acute experimental torsion of the spermatic cord. AJR Am J Roentgenol. 1996 Sep;167(3):785-90. doi: 10.2214/ajr.167.3.8751701. PMID: 8751701.

57- Cimador M, DiPace MR, Castagnetti M, DeGrazia E. Predictors of testicular viability in testicular torsion. J Pediatr Urol. 2007 Oct;3(5):387-90. doi: 10.1016/j.jpurol.2007.01.194. Epub 2007 Apr 2. PMID: 18947779.

58- Bolln C, Driver CP, Youngson GG. Operative management of testicular torsion: current practice within the UK and Ireland. J Pediatr Urol. 2006 Jun;2(3):190-3. doi: 10.1016/j.jpurol.2005.07.006. Epub 2005 Aug 31. PMID: 18947607.

59- Gesino A, Bachmann De Santos ME. Spermatic cord torsion after testicular fixation. A different surgical approach and a revision of current techniques. Eur J Pediatr Surg. 2001 Dec;11(6):404-10. doi: 10.1055/s-2001-19721. PMID: 11807671.

60- I. Duquesne, U. Pinar, F. Bardet, I. Dominique, K. Kaulanjan, X. Matillon, C. Michiels, M. Vallée, Z. Khene, B. Pradère.CONTROLATERAL ORCHIDOPEXY DURING SCROTAL EXPLORATION FOR SUSPICION OF TORSION: IS IT REALLY SAFE? RISK ?. Prog Urol, 2020, 13, 30, 727

61- Cattolica EV, Karol JB, Rankin KN, Klein RS. High testicular salvage rate in torsion of the spermatic cord. J Urol. 1982 Jul;128(1):66-8. doi: 10.1016/s0022-5347(17)52758-5. PMID: 7109074.

APPENDIXES

APPENDIX 1

NAME :

FIRST NAME :

Age (in months):

Month of consultation:

Family history: cryptorchidism

Personal history: prematurity, low birth weight, omphalocele or other abdominal wall anomaly inguinal hernia

Comorbidities: microcephaly, epilepsy, BMI, mental retardation, spastic quadriplegia, down syndrome, spastic neuromuscular disease, neuromuscular scoliosis, congenital hip dysplasia, posterior vertebral fusion, necrotizing enterocolitis, GERD, pellagra encephalopathy (vit B deficiency).

Symptomatology :

Duration of symptoms: (in hours)

Associated signs: nausea, vomiting, fever, urinary signs Physical examination :
Elements: Governor's sign; infiltrated cord, absent cremasteric reflex, negative prehn's sign, local inflammatory signs, low sensitivity.

side: (right or left testicle affected)

Radiology: Doppler ultrasound (timing in relation to consultation and symptomatology)

MRI scintigraphy

Anomalies described :

Biology: inflammatory and infectious work-up (CBC - CRP)

Location of the affected testicle

Degree of testicular torsion: (number of turns) Manual detorsion manoeuvre carried out or not

Surgery :

Inguinal or scrotal approach Intraoperative findings Orchidectomy or fixation procedures

Contralateral testis: location and fixation Post-operatively :

Complications

Anatomopathological examination for orchiectomy Duration of post-operative follow-up :

Step back

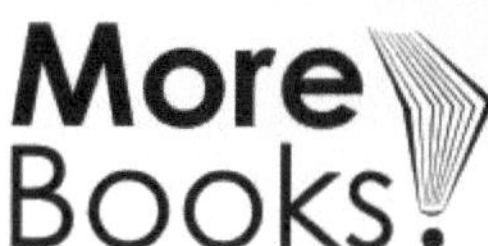

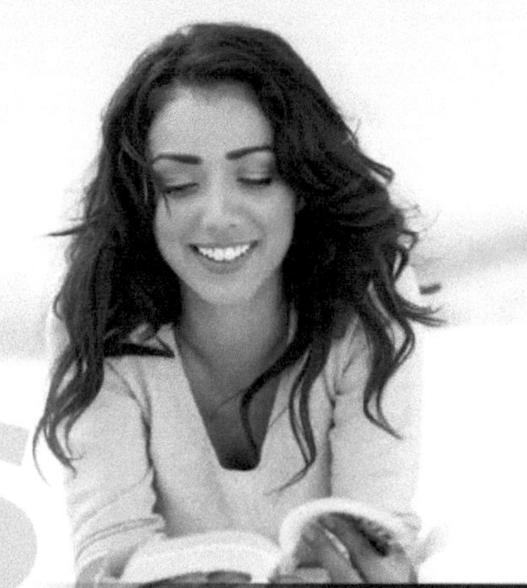

yes

I want morebooks!

Buy your books fast and straightforward online - at one of world's fastest growing online book stores! Environmentally sound due to Print-on-Demand technologies.

Buy your books online at

www.morebooks.shop

Kaufen Sie Ihre Bücher schnell und unkompliziert online – auf einer der am schnellsten wachsenden Buchhandelsplattformen weltweit! Dank Print-On-Demand umwelt- und ressourcenschonend produzi ert.

Bücher schneller online kaufen

www.morebooks.shop

info@omniscriptum.com
www.omniscriptum.com

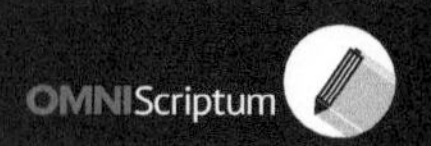

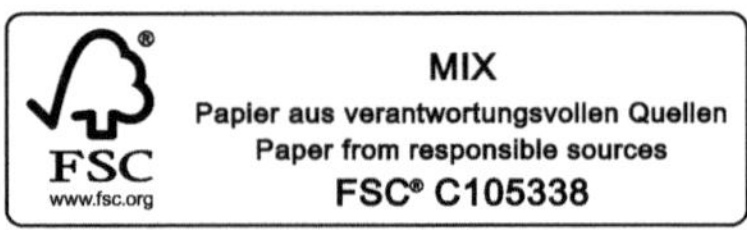

Printed by Books on Demand GmbH, Norderstedt / Germany